Man...
severe and
complicated malaria

A practical handbook

H. M. Gilles
Emeritus Professor of Tropical Medicine
Liverpool School of Tropical Medicine
University of Liverpool
Liverpool, England

*Based on: Severe and complicated malaria, 2nd ed.,
edited by D. A. Warrell, M. E. Molyneux & P. F. Beales
(Transactions of the Royal Society of Tropical Medicine
and Hygiene, 1990, 84 (Suppl. 2))*

World Health Organization
Geneva 1991

Reprinted 1993, 1995, 1997, 1998

WHO Library Cataloguing in Publication Data

Gilles, H. M.
   Management of severe and complicated malaria: a practical
   handbook / H. M. Gilles.

   1. Malaria – complications – handbooks 2. Malaria – therapy –
   handbooks I. Title

   ISBN 92 4 154436 8   (NLM Classification: WC 39)

DESIGNED BY WHO GRAPHICS
PRINTED IN ENGLAND
91/ 8900 – 93 / 9713 – 95 / 10433 – 96 / 11165 – 16000
97 / 11644 – GR – 2500

■ Contents

◼ Preface

Malaria continues to be a major global health problem, with over 40% of the world's population — more than 2000 million people — exposed to varying degrees of malaria risk in some 100 countries. In addition, with modern rapid means of travel, large numbers of people from nonmalarious areas are being exposed to infection which may only seriously affect them after they have returned home

Plasmodium falciparum causes the most serious form of the disease, and is common in the tropics. Infections with this parasite can be fatal in the absence of prompt recognition of the disease and its complications, and active appropriate patient management. The situation is complicated by the increasing occurrence of *P. falciparum* parasites that are resistant to chloroquine and other antimalarial drugs. Prompt action is especially important for high-risk groups such as young children and pregnant women.

Because of the increasing seriousness of this problem, the World Health Organization invited Professor H. M. Gilles to prepare this *aide-mémoire* on the clinical diagnosis and management of severe malaria. It is intended primarily for physicians and other responsible health personnel working in hospitals, or health centres with inpatient facilities, in malarious areas of the world, but will also be of practical use to physicians in nonendemic countries.

This handbook is based on "Severe and complicated malaria", edited by D. A. Warrell, M. E. Molyneux and P. F. Beales, and published in *Transactions of the Royal Society of Tropical Medicine and Hygiene*, 1990, 84 (Suppl 2). During the preparation of this guide, valuable advice was provided by a number of colleagues. Professor Gilles and the World Health Organization gratefully acknowledge the very willing collaboration and support given by Professor D. A. Warrell, Nuffield Department of Clinical Medicine, University of Oxford; Dr M. E. Molyneux, Liverpool School of Tropical Medicine; Professor Tan Chongsupphajaisiddhi, School of Tropical Medicine, Bangkok; Professor Khunying Tranachit Harinasuta, Bangkok; Professor Looareesuwan, Hospital for Tropical Diseases, Bangkok; Dr N. J. White, Wellcome–Mahidol University–Oxford Tropical Medical Research Programme; Dr A. P. Hall, Hospital for Tropical Diseases, London; Dr R. N. Davidson, Hospital for Tropical Diseases, London; and Dr P. F. Beales and Dr R. Kouznetsov, Training Unit, Division of Control of Tropical Diseases, World Health Organization, Geneva.

■ Introduction

Severe and complicated malaria is caused by *Plasmodium falciparum* infection (Fig. 1). It occurs almost invariably as a result of delay in treating an uncomplicated attack, because of misdiagnosis or for other reasons, but occasionally may develop very rapidly.

The presentation of uncomplicated *P. falciparum* malaria is very variable and mimics that of many other diseases. Although fever is very common, it is absent in some cases. The fever is initially persistent rather than tertian (Fig. 2) and may or may not be accompanied by rigors.

The patient commonly complains of fever, headache, and aches and pains elsewhere over the body; on physical examination the liver and spleen may be palpable. This clinical presentation in nonendemic or low-endemic areas may be misdiagnosed as influenza. Abdominal pain and diarrhoea are inconsistently complained of. Unless diagnosed and treated promptly the clinical picture deteriorates at an alarming speed and often with catastrophic consequences.

Fig. 1. **Global status of** *P. falciparum* **malaria**

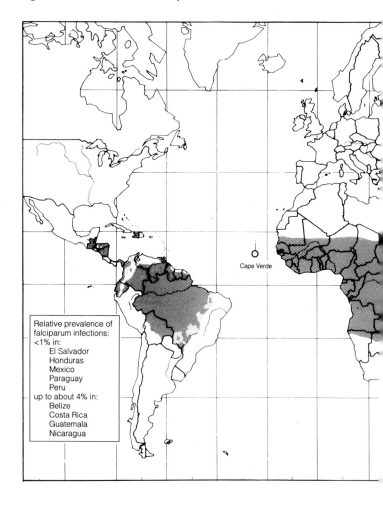

Cape Verde

Relative prevalence of
falciparum infections:
<1% in:
    El Salvador
    Honduras
    Mexico
    Paraguay
    Peru
up to about 4% in:
    Belize
    Costa Rica
    Guatemala
    Nicaragua

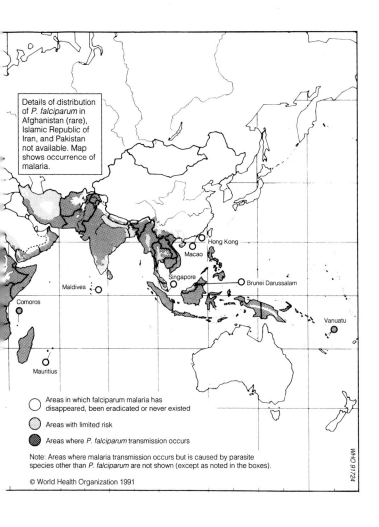

Details of distribution of *P. falciparum* in Afghanistan (rare), Islamic Republic of Iran, and Pakistan not available. Map shows occurrence of malaria.

Hong Kong

Macao

Singapore

Brunei Darussalam

Maldives

Comoros

Vanuatu

Mauritius

○ Areas in which falciparum malaria has disappeared, been eradicated or never existed

◐ Areas with limited risk

● Areas where *P. falciparum* transmission occurs

Note: Areas where malaria transmission occurs but is caused by parasite species other than *P. falciparum* are not shown (except as noted in the boxes).

© World Health Organization 1991

WHO 91724

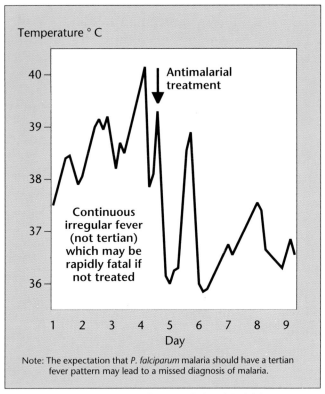

Fig. 2. **Temperature chart characteristic of *P. falciparum* malaria**

Severe and complicated malaria

A patient with severe and complicated malaria may present with impaired consciousness (but be rousable), prostration and extreme weakness, and jaundice. In addition, the following complications may occur:

- Cerebral malaria, defined as unrousable coma not attributable to any other cause in a patient with falciparum malaria.

- Generalized convulsions.

- Normocytic anaemia.

- Renal failure.

- Hypoglycaemia.

- Fluid, electrolyte and acid–base disturbances.

- Pulmonary oedema.

- Circulatory collapse and shock ("algid malaria").

- Spontaneous bleeding (disseminated intravascular coagulation).

- Hyperpyrexia.

- Hyperparasitaemia.

- Malarial haemoglobinuria.

It is important to appreciate that these severe manifestations can occur singly, or more commonly in combination in the same patient. Children and nonimmune adults are at most risk in endemic areas.

General management

The following measures should be applied to all patients with clinically diagnosed or suspected severe malaria:

- If parasitological confirmation of malaria is not readily available, a blood film should be made and treatment started on the basis of the clinical presentation.

- Antimalarial chemotherapy must be given parenterally (intravenously or intramuscularly). Oral treatment should be substituted as soon as reliably possible.

- Doses must be calculated on a mg/kg of body weight basis. It is therefore important whenever possible to weigh the patient. This is particularly important for children.

- Do not confuse the doses of salt and base. Quinine doses are usually prescribed as salt (10 mg of salt = 8.3 mg of base). Chloroquine, quinidine and mefloquine are commonly prescribed as base.

- Good nursing care is vital (see page 9).

- If an intensive care unit is available, patients should be admitted to it.

- If fluids are being given intravenously, careful attention to fluid balance is important in order to avoid overhydration and underhydration.

- A rapid initial check of blood glucose level and frequent monitoring for hypoglycaemia are important, when possible; otherwise glucose should be given.

- Unconscious patients should receive meticulous nursing care (see page 9). Indwelling urinary catheters should be removed as soon as they are no longer necessary or if the patient becomes anuric.

- Other treatable causes of coma should be excluded (by lumbar puncture) or covered by treatment (see pages 17–18 and 22).

- Frequent monitoring of the therapeutic response, both parasitaemic and clinical, is important .

- Look for and manage any complicating or associated infections.

- Monitor urine output constantly and look for the appearance of black urine (see pages 16–17 and 25–26).

- Regular monitoring of the core temperature, respiration rate, blood pressure, level of consciousness and other vital signs is mandatory.

- Reduce high body temperatures (>39 °C) by vigorous tepid sponging and fanning. Antipyretics may also be given (see pages 9, 24 and 29).

- Blood cultures should be taken if the patient goes into shock while undergoing treatment.

- Laboratory measurements should include regular checks on erythrocyte volume fraction (haematocrit), glucose, urea or creatinine, and electrolytes.

- Initial ophthalmoscopic examination of the fundus is important, since the presence of retinal haemorrhages has diagnostic and prognostic significance in some areas of the world (Fig. 3).

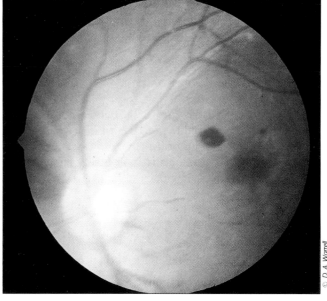

© D. A. Warrell

Fig. 3. **Two retinal haemorrhages close to the macula in a Thai patient with cerebral malaria**

- Administer a prophylactic anticonvulsant, e.g. phenobarbital sodium, 10–15 mg/kg of body weight, by intramuscular injection.

- Drugs that increase the risk of gastrointestinal bleeding (aspirin, corticosteroids) should be avoided as far as possible.

More sophisticated monitoring may be useful if complications develop, and will depend on the local availability of equipment, experience and skills. Insertion sites for intravenous lines should be cleaned at least twice daily with iodine and alcohol.

Nursing care

The management of the patient with severe malaria is as important as chemotherapy and here the nurse has a crucial role to play.

- Meticulous nursing care should be given to unconscious patients. Maintain a clear airway. Turn the patient every two hours. Do not allow the patient to lie in a wet bed. Particular attention should be paid to pressure points and the patient should be nursed on his or her side to avoid aspiration of fluid. Aspiration pneumonia is a potentially fatal complication, and must be dealt with immediately (see inside back cover flap).

- A careful record of fluid intake and output must be kept, the appearance of black urine noted and specific gravity measured.

- The speed of infusion of fluids should be checked frequently.

- Temperature, pulse, respiration and blood pressure must be monitored regularly every 4–6 hours for at least the first 48 hours.

- Changes in the level of consciousness, occurrence of convulsions or changes in behaviour of the patient must be reported immediately.

- If rectal temperature rises above 39 °C, vigorous tepid sponging and fanning must be applied, and paracetamol may be given.

Specific antimalarial chemotherapy

The drugs appropriate for the treatment of severe falciparum malaria are given in Table 1 on the inside front cover flap. Information on the most commonly used drugs is given in Annex 1. Response should be monitored by frequent clinical examination including recording of fluid balance, temperature, pulse, blood pressure, jugular venous pressure, and parasitaemia (in blood films) every 4–6 hours for the first 48 hours.

The global status of chloroquine resistance is shown in the map on the inside back cover. A comparison of this map with that in Fig. 1 clearly indicates that there is hardly a malaria-endemic country where resistance of *P. falciparum* to chloroquine has not been reported.

■ Salient clinical features
■ and management of
■ complications

In all cases of severe malaria, parenteral antimalarial chemotherapy should be started immediately. Any complications can then be dealt with as described below.

Cerebral malaria

Clinical features

The patient with cerebral malaria is comatose, the depth of consciousness being variable (for assessment of coma, see Glasgow coma scale in Annex 2). If in doubt as to cause, test for other locally prevalent encephalopathies, e.g. bacterial and fungal meningoencephalitides and viral encephalitides. Asexual malaria parasites are usually demonstrable on a peripheral blood smear. Convulsions are common in both adults and children. Retinal haemorrhages are associated with a poor prognosis in adults (Fig. 3); papilloedema is rare. A variety of transient abnormalities of eye movement, especially disconjugate gaze, have been noted (Fig. 4). Fixed jaw closure and tooth grinding (bruxism) are common. Pouting may occur (Fig. 5) or a pout reflex may be elicited (by stroking the sides of the mouth). Mild neck stiffness occurs but neck rigidity and photophobia are absent. The commonest neurological picture in adults is one of a symmetrical upper motor neuron lesion. The duration of coma varies from about 6 to 96 hours in adults.

Motor abnormalities such as decerebrate rigidity (Fig. 6), decorticate rigidity (arms flexed and legs stretched), and opisthotonos (Fig. 7) occur. The opening pressure at lumbar puncture is usually normal in adults, but may be elevated; the

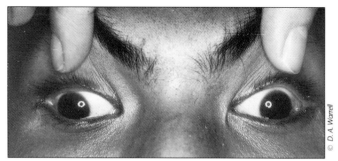

Fig. 4. **Disconjugate gaze in a Thai man with cerebral malaria: optic axes are nonparallel in vertical and horizontal planes**

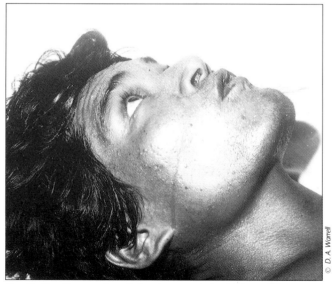

Fig. 5. **Pouting and sustained upward deviation of the eyes accompanied by laboured and noisy breathing in a Thai man with cerebral malaria complicated by hypoglycaemia**

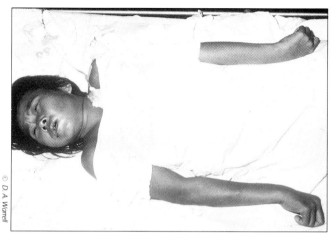

Fig. 6. **Decerebrate rigidity in a Thai woman with cerebral malaria complicated by hypoglycaemia**

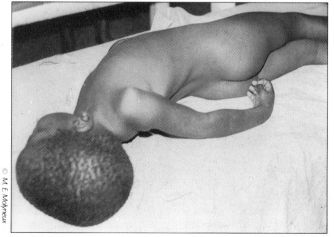

Fig. 7. **Opisthotonos in an unrousably comatose child with cerebral malaria. The cerebrospinal fluid cell count was normal**

cerebrospinal fluid (CSF) is clear, with fewer than 10 white cells per μl; the protein is raised as is the CSF lactic acid concentration. A variety of nonspecific electroencephalogram (EEG) abnormalities have been described; computerized tomography scans of the brain are usually normal. Hepatosplenomegaly is common. The abdominal reflexes are invariably absent; this is a useful sign for distinguishing hysterical adult patients with fevers of other causes, in whom these reflexes are usually brisk.

See pages 29–30 for a description of the clinical features of cerebral malaria in children.

Management

- The comatose patient should be given meticulous nursing care (see page 9).

- Insert a urethral catheter using a sterile technique, unless the patient is anuric.

- Keep an accurate record of fluid intake and output.

- Monitor and record the level of consciousness (using the Glasgow coma scale, Annex 2), temperature, respiratory rate, blood pressure, and vital signs.

- Give a single intramuscular injection of phenobarbital sodium, 10–15 mg/kg of body weight, to prevent convulsions.

- Treat convulsions if and when they arise with diazepam or paraldehyde. A slow intravenous injection of diazepam (0.15 mg/kg of body weight, maximum 10 mg for adults) or intramuscular injection of paraldehyde (0.1 ml/kg of body weight, from a glass syringe) will usually control convulsions. Diazepam can also be given intrarectally (0.5–1.0 mg/kg of body weight) if injection is not possible.

Avoid the following:

— corticosteroids,
— other anti-inflammatory agents,
— other agents given for cerebral oedema (urea, invert sugar),
— low molecular weight dextran,
— epinephrine (adrenaline),
— heparin,
— epoprostenol (prostacyclin),
— pentoxifylline (oxpentifylline),
— hyperbaric oxygen,
— ciclosporin (cyclosporin A).

Anaemia

Clinical features

Anaemia is common in severe malaria. In African children, anaemia is a common presenting feature; parasitaemia is often low but there is abundant malarial pigment in monocytes and other phagocytic cells, reflecting recent or resolving infection. This presentation in non-African children is less well recognized.

Anaemia is often associated with secondary bacterial infection, retinal haemorrhage and pregnancy.

Management

- If the haematocrit falls below 20%, give a transfusion of pathogen-free compatible fresh blood or packed cells. (Stored bank blood may be used if fresh blood is not available.) In areas where human immunodeficiency virus (HIV) is prevalent and facilities for screening are inadequate, the general condition of the patient (e.g. shock, cardiac failure) and the response to oxygen and colloid infusion should be the guiding principles rather than the haematocrit alone.

- Provided that the patient's renal function is adequate, give small intravenous doses of furosemide 20 mg during the blood transfusion as necessary to avoid circulatory overload.

- Remember to include the volume of transfused cells or blood in calculations of fluid balance.

Renal failure

Clinical features

Renal failure as a complication of malaria is virtually confined to adults. There is a rise in serum creatinine and urea, oliguria and eventually anuria due to acute tubular necrosis. Renal failure is usually oliguric but may occasionally be polyuric. The mechanism of acute tubular necrosis in malaria is not fully understood. Studies of renal blood flow have shown cortical ischaemia and medullary congestion as in other forms of acute tubular necrosis.

Acute renal failure is usually reversible.

Management

- Exclude dehydration (hypovolaemia) by clinical examination, including measurement of jugular or central venous pressure, and blood pressure drop between the patient lying supine and when propped up to 45°.

- Carefully infuse isotonic saline until venous pressure is between 0 and 5 cm H_2O (Annex 3).

- Peritoneal dialysis or haemodialysis is indicated if the patient remains oliguric after adequate rehydration and the blood urea and creatinine rise progressively.

- Peritoneal dialysis should not be undertaken lightly. If possible, refer the patient to a dialysis unit or centre.

Hypoglycaemia

Clinical features

Hypoglycaemia is increasingly being recognized as an important manifestation of falciparum malaria. It occurs in three different groups of patients which may overlap:

- patients with severe disease, especially young children (see page 32);

- patients treated with quinine or quinidine, as a result of a quinine-induced hyperinsulinaemia;

- pregnant women, either on admission or following quinine treatment (see pages 36–37).

In conscious patients, hypoglycaemia may present with classic symptoms of anxiety, sweating, dilatation of the pupils, breathlessness, laboured and noisy breathing, oliguria, a feeling of coldness, tachycardia and light-headedness. This clinical picture may develop into deteriorating consciousness, generalized convulsions, extensor posturing, shock and coma.

The diagnosis is easily overlooked because all these clinical features also occur in severe malaria itself. A deterioration in the level of consciousness may be the only sign. If possible, confirm by biochemical testing, especially in the high-risk groups mentioned above.

Management

- If hypoglycaemia is detected by blood testing or suspected on clinical grounds, give 50% glucose, 50 ml (1.0 ml/kg for children) by intravenous bolus injection.

- Follow with an intravenous infusion of 5% or 10% glucose.

- Continue to monitor blood glucose levels (using a "stix" method if available, or clinically and biochemically if not) in order to regulate the glucose infusion. Remember that hypoglycaemia may recur even after an intravenous bolus of 50% glucose.

Fluid, electrolyte and acid–base disturbances

Clinical features

Patients with severe falciparum malaria often show the following on admission: clinical evidence of *hypovolaemia* — low jugular venous pressure, postural hypotension, and oliguria with high urine specific gravity; and clinical signs of *dehydration* — reduced ocular tension and decreased skin turgor.

Acidotic breathing—hyperventilation—may develop in severely ill patients who are shocked, hypoglycaemic, hyperparasitaemic, or in renal failure. Lactic acidosis is a common complication and both blood and CSF lactic acid concentrations are raised. Perfusion is improved by correcting hypovolaemia.

Management

- Look for evidence of dehydration and hypovolaemia:

  — reduced ocular tension,
  — reduced skin turgor,
  — relatively cool extremities,
  — postural drop in blood pressure (as the patient is propped up from the lying-down position to 45°),
  — reduced peripheral venous filling,
  — low jugular venous pressure,
  — reduced urine output,
  — high urine specific gravity,
  — urine sodium concentration less than 20 mmol/l.

- If there is evidence of dehydration, give modest volumes of isotonic fluids (0.9% saline or 5% dextrose) by intravenous infusion, but avoid fluid overload.

- Monitor blood pressure, urine volume (every hour), and jugular or central venous pressure (Annex 3).

- Improve oxygenation by

  — clearing airway,
  — increasing concentration of inspired oxygen, and
  — supporting ventilation artificially, if necessary.

Pulmonary oedema

Clinical features

Pulmonary oedema is a grave complication of severe malaria, with a high mortality (over 50%). It may appear several days after chemotherapy has been started and at a time when the patient's general condition is improving and the peripheral parasitaemia is diminishing. It must be differentiated from iatrogenically produced pulmonary oedema resulting from fluid overload. Hyperparasitaemia, renal failure and pregnancy (see page 37) are often associated, as well as hypoglycaemia and metabolic acidosis. The first indication of impending pulmonary oedema is an increase in the respiratory rate, which precedes the development of other chest signs (Fig. 8).

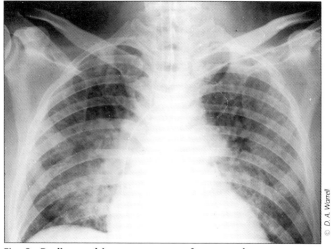

© D. A. Warrell

Fig. 8. **Radiographic appearances of acute pulmonary oedema, resembling adult respiratory distress syndrome, in a British patient with cerebral malaria**

Hypoxia may cause convulsions and deterioration in the level of consciousness and the patient may die within a few hours.

Management

- Keep patient upright; raise the head of the bed or lower the foot of the bed.

- Give a high concentration of oxygen by any convenient method available, including mechanical ventilation.

- Give the patient a diuretic, such as furosemide 40 mg, by intravenous injection. If there is no response, increase the dose progressively to a maximum of 200 mg.

- In well-equipped intensive care units, mechanical ventilation with positive end expiratory pressure (PEEP), a wide range of vasoactive drugs and haemodynamic monitoring will be available.

If the pulmonary oedema is due to overhydration:

- Stop all intravenous fluids.

- Use haemofiltration immediately, if available.

- Give furosemide 40 mg intravenously. If there is no response, increase the dose progressively to a maximum of 200 mg.

- If there is no improvement, withdraw 250 ml of blood initially by venesection into a blood transfusion donor bag so that it can be given back to the patient later.

Circulatory collapse ("algid malaria")

Clinical features

Some patients are admitted in a state of collapse, with a systolic blood pressure less than 80 mmHg in the supine position (less than 50 mmHg in children); a cold, clammy, cyanotic skin; constricted peripheral veins; rapid feeble pulse. In some countries this clinical picture is often associated with a complicating Gram-negative septicaemia.

Circulatory collapse is also seen in patients with pulmonary oedema or metabolic acidosis, and following massive gastrointestinal haemorrhage. Dehydration with hypovolaemia may also contribute to hypotension.

Possible sites of associated infection should be sought, e.g. lung, urinary tract (especially if there is an indwelling catheter), meningitis, intravenous injection sites, intravenous lines.

Management

- Correct hypovolaemia with an appropriate plasma expander (fresh blood, plasma, polygeline or dextran 70).

- Take a blood culture and start patient on broad-spectrum antibiotics immediately, e.g. combined treatment with benzylpenicillin and gentamicin.

- Once the results of blood culture and sensitivity testing are available, give the appropriate antibiotic.

- Maintain central venous pressure between 0 and 5 cm H_2O (see Annex 3; if hypotension persists dopamine may be given through a central line).

Spontaneous bleeding and disseminated intravascular coagulation

Clinical features

Bleeding gums, epistaxis, petechiae, and subconjunctival haemorrhages may occur (Fig. 9). Disseminated intravascular coagulation, complicated by clinically significant bleeding, e.g. haematemesis or melaena, occurs in fewer than 10% of patients; it seems to occur more often in nonimmune patients. It is relatively common in nonimmune patients with imported malaria in the temperate zone. Thrombocytopenia is common, and is not related to other measures of coagulation or to plasma fibrinogen concentrations; in most cases it is

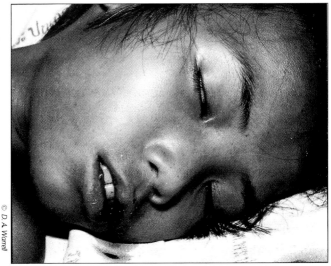

© D. A. Warrell

Fig. 9. **Profound anaemia, cerebral malaria, disseminated intravascular coagulation and spontaneous bleeding from the gums in a Thai girl**

unaccompanied by bleeding. The platelet count usually returns to normal after successful treatment of the malaria.

Management

- Transfuse fresh blood, clotting factors or platelets as required.

- If the prothrombin or partial thromboplastin times are prolonged, give vitamin K, 10 mg, by slow intravenous injection.

Hyperpyrexia

Clinical features

Hyperpyrexia is more common in children and is associated with convulsions, delirium, and coma. In unacclimatized visitors to the tropics, it must be differentiated from heat stroke.

High body temperatures (42 °C and above) may cause permanent severe neurological sequelae. There is evidence that high body temperature in pregnant women contributes to fetal distress (see page 36).

Management

- Monitor rectal temperature frequently.

- If rectal temperature is above 39 °C, apply vigorous tepid sponging and fanning, and give paracetamol, 15 mg/kg of body weight by mouth, suppository or nasogastric tube.

Hyperparasitaemia

Clinical features

In general, and especially in nonimmune subjects, high parasite densities (above 5%) and peripheral schizontaemia are associated with severe disease; however, in highly endemic malarious areas, partially immune children can tolerate surprisingly high densities (20–30%) often without clinical symptoms.

Management

- An initial dose of parenteral antimalarial therapy (see Table 1, inside front cover flap) is prudent, even if the patient can take medication by mouth.

- Some physicians recommend exchange or partial exchange transfusion (between quinine infusions) if parasitaemia exceeds 10% in a severely ill patient.

- The risks of the above procedures in the tropics, e.g. from transfusion-related infections and incurred risk of bacterial infection, must be carefully assessed.

Malarial haemoglobinuria

Clinical features

Patients with glucose-6-phosphate dehydrogenase deficiency and some other erythrocyte enzyme deficiencies may develop vascular haemolysis and haemoglobinuria when treated with oxidant drugs such as primaquine, even in the absence of malaria. "Blackwater fever" — which typically occurred in nonimmune Caucasian patients taking quinine irregularly for prophylaxis or presumptive treatment, was accompanied by mild or absent fever, scanty or absent parasitaemia, and carried a poor prognosis — is now very rare.

Malarial haemoglobinuria is uncommon and is usually associated with hyperparasitaemia and/or severe disease. It may or may not be accompanied by renal failure. The patient is anaemic.

Management

- Continue appropriate antimalarial treatment (see Table 1, inside front cover flap) if parasitaemia is present.

- Transfuse fresh blood to maintain haematocrit above 20%.

- Monitor jugular or central venous pressure to avoid fluid overload and hypovolaemia (Annex 3).

- Give furosemide 20 mg intravenously.

- If oliguria develops and blood urea and serum creatinine levels rise, peritoneal dialysis or haemodialysis may be required.

Special clinical features of severe malaria and management of common complications in children

Severe malaria

Clinical features

Many of the clinical features of severe malaria described on pages 11–26 also occur in children. Only certain additional points will be highlighted here. The commonest and most important complications of *P. falciparum* infection in children are cerebral malaria and severe anaemia.

The differences between severe malaria in adults and in children are given in Table 2.

Management

The management of severe malaria in children is generally similar to that in adults (see pages 11–26). Some specific aspects will be re-emphasized here.

- The parents or other relatives should be questioned about: (i) history of residence or travel; (ii) previous treatment with antimalarials or other drugs; (iii) recent fluid intake and urine output; and (iv) recent or past history of convulsions.

- A rapid initial examination should be carried out to assess: (i) hydration; (ii) anaemia; (iii) pulmonary oedema; (iv) level of consciousness; and (v) hyperpyrexia.

(continued overleaf)

Table 2 **Differences between severe malaria in adults and in children[a]**

Sign or symptom	Adults	Children
Cough	Uncommon	Common
Convulsions	Common	Very common
Duration of illness	5–7 days	1–2 days
Resolution of coma	2–4 days	1–2 days
Neurological sequelae	< 5%	> 10%
Jaundice	Common	Uncommon
Pretreatment hypoglycaemia	Uncommon	Common
Pulmonary oedema	Common	Rare
Renal failure	Common	Rare
CSF opening pressure	Usually normal	Variable, often raised
Bleeding/clotting disturbances	Up to 10%	Rare
Abnormality of brain stem reflexes (e.g. oculovestibular, oculocervical).	Rare	More common

[a] Derived from studies in South-East Asian adults and African children.

- Immediate tests must include: (i) thick and thin blood films; (ii) haematocrit; (iii) finger-prick blood glucose; and (iv) lumbar puncture.

- If parasitological confirmation is likely to take more than one hour, treatment should be started before the diagnosis is confirmed.

- The use of a single intramuscular injection of phenobarbital sodium 10–15 mg/kg of body weight on admission may reduce the incidence of convulsions.

- If the child has a convulsion, this should be treated with paraldehyde 0.1 mg/kg of body weight intramuscularly. Ideally, a glass syringe should be used, but a plastic syringe is satisfactory provided the injection is given immediately after the drug has been drawn into the syringe. Diazepam may also be used (page 14).

- Any child with convulsions should be examined for hyperpyrexia and hypoglycaemia and given appropriate treatment.

- Simple practical manoeuvres, such as tepid sponging and fanning, should be employed to try to keep the rectal temperature below 39 °C. Relatives are usually happy to do this when instructed.

- Paracetamol, 15 mg/kg of body weight, may also be given as an antipyretic.

Cerebral malaria (see also pages 11–15)

Clinical features

- The earliest symptom of cerebral malaria in children is usually fever (37.5–41 °C), followed by failure to eat or drink. Vomiting and cough are common; diarrhoea is unusual.

- The history of symptoms preceding coma may be very brief — commonly one or two days.

- A child who loses consciousness after a febrile convulsion should not be considered to have cerebral malaria unless coma persists for more than half an hour after the convulsion.

- The depth of coma may be assessed according to the Glasgow coma scale, by observing the response to standard vocal or painful stimuli (rub knuckles on child's sternum; if no response, apply firm pressure on thumbnail bed with horizontal pencil).

- Always exclude or treat hypoglycaemia (see page 32).

- Convulsions are common before or after the onset of coma. They are significantly associated with morbidity and sequelae.

- In some children the breathing is laboured and noisy; in others, deep breathing with a clear chest suggests acidosis.

- A few children have cold, clammy skin, with a core-to-skin temperature difference of 10 °C. Some of these patients are in a state of shock with a systolic blood pressure below 50 mmHg.

- In patients with profound coma, corneal reflexes and "doll's eye" movements may be absent.

- In some children, extreme opisthotonos is seen (Fig. 7, p.13), which may lead to a mistaken diagnosis of tetanus or meningitis.

- CSF opening pressure is variable; it is raised more frequently than in adults, and is sometimes very high.

- Leukocytosis is not unusual in severe disease and does not necessarily imply an associated bacterial infection. (This is also true in adults.)

- A proportion of children (about 10%) who survive cerebral malaria have neurological sequelae which persist into the convalescent period. Sequelae may take the form of hemiparesis, cerebellar ataxia, cortical blindness, severe hypotonia, mental retardation, generalized spasticity, or aphasia.

Management

The management of cerebral malaria in children is the same as for adults (see page 14).

Anaemia

Clinical features

The rate of development and degree of anaemia depend on the severity and duration of parasitaemia. In some children, repeated untreated episodes of otherwise uncomplicated malaria may lead to normochromic anaemia in which dyserythropoietic changes in the bone marrow are prominent. Parasitaemia is often scanty, although numerous pigmented monocytes can be seen in the peripheral blood.

In other children, severe anaemia may develop rapidly in association with hyperparasitaemia. In these cases, acute destruction of parasitized red cells is responsible.

Children with severe anaemia may present with tachycardia and dyspnoea. Anaemia may contribute both to *cerebral signs* — confusion, restlessness, coma and retinal haemorrhages — and to *cardiopulmonary signs* — gallop rhythm, cardiac failure, hepatomegaly and pulmonary oedema.

Management

- The need for blood transfusion must be assessed with great care in each individual child. Not only the level of the haematocrit, but the density of parasitaemia and the clinical condition of the patient must be taken into account.

- In general and with the proviso mentioned above, a haematocrit of less than 15% in a normally hydrated child is an indication for blood transfusion. In some children, an initial transfusion is required with the utmost urgency (10 ml of packed cells or 20 ml of whole blood per kg of body weight).

- If HIV-screened blood is not available, fresh blood from an elderly relative is preferable for transfusion as it decreases the risk of HIV infection.

- Furosemide, 1–2 mg/kg of body weight up to a maximum of 20 mg, may be given intravenously to avoid fluid overload.

Hypoglycaemia

Clinical features

Hypoglycaemia is particularly common in young children (under 3 years), in those with convulsions or hyperparasitaemia, and in patients with profound coma. It is easily overlooked clinically because the manifestations may be similar to those of cerebral malaria (see also pages 17–18).

Management

- Unconscious children should be given glucose regularly to prevent starvation hypoglycaemia. It is most conveniently provided as 5% dextrose in water infusion, but if this would be likely to lead to fluid overload, smaller volumes of more concentrated glucose may be given at regular intervals.

- If hypoglycaemia occurs, it should be treated with an intravenous bolus injection of 50% glucose (up to 1.0 ml/kg of body weight) followed by a slow intravenous infusion of 10% glucose to prevent recurrence of hypoglycaemia. The duration and amount of glucose infusion will be dictated by the results of blood glucose monitoring (which should be done in blood taken from the arm opposite to that receiving the infusion), using a "stix" method.

- Monitoring of blood glucose levels should continue even after apparent recovery, since hypoglycaemia may recur.

Dehydration

Clinical features

The best clinical indications of mild to moderate dehydration in children are decreased peripheral perfusion, deep (acidotic) breathing, decreased skin turgor, raised blood urea (>6.5 mmol/l), increased thirst, loss of about 3–4% of total body weight and evidence of metabolic acidosis.

In children presenting with oliguria and dehydration, examination of urine usually reveals a high specific gravity, low urinary sodium, and a normal urinary sediment, indicating simple dehydration rather than renal failure, which is rare in children.

Management

- Careful rehydration with isotonic saline is mandatory, with frequent examination of the jugular venous pressure, blood pressure and chest.

- Where facilities for monitoring and maintenance of adequate sterility exist, fluid balance may be adjusted in accordance with direct measurement of the central venous pressure through a central venous catheter (Annex 3).

- If, after careful rehydration, urine output over 24 hours is less than 4 ml/kg of body weight, furosemide can be given intravenously, initially at 2 mg/kg of body weight, then doubled at hourly intervals to a maximum of 8 mg/kg of body weight (given over 15 minutes).

Antimalarial drugs
(see Table 1 inside front cover flap and Annex 1)

Antimalarial drugs should preferably be given initially by intravenous infusion; this should be replaced by oral administration as soon as possible.

Weighing of children is mandatory and the dose of antimalarials should be calculated on the basis of body weight (mg/kg) (Table 1).

If intravenous infusion is not possible, chloroquine and quinine may be given by intramuscular injection into the anterior thigh. Chloroquine — but not quinine — may also be given by subcutaneous injection.

Do not attempt to give oral medication to unconscious children; if parenteral injection is not possible and referral is likely to be delayed, antimalarials may be given by nasogastric tube. However, nasogastric administration may cause vomiting and produce inadequate drug levels in the blood.

■ Special clinical features
■ and management of severe
■ malaria in pregnancy

Severe malaria

Clinical features

Pregnant women with malaria must be treated promptly, because the disease is more severe, is associated with high parasitaemia, and is dangerous for mother and fetus.

Nonimmune pregnant women are susceptible to all the manifestations described on pages 11–26. Moreover they have an increased risk of abortion, stillbirth, premature delivery and

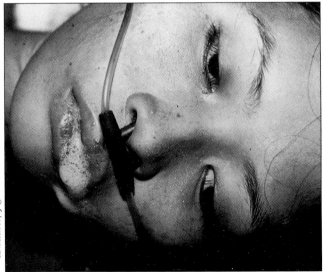

Fig. 10. **Acute pulmonary oedema developing immediately after delivery in a Thai woman**

low birth weight of their infant. They are more likely to develop cerebral and other forms of severe malaria, and to suffer a high mortality — 2–10 times higher than nonpregnant patients. They are particularly susceptible to hypoglycaemia and acute pulmonary oedema (Fig. 10).

Partially immune pregnant women, especially primigravidae, are susceptible to severe anaemia but other complications are unusual.

Falciparum malaria commonly induces uterine contractions and gives rise to premature labour. The frequency and intensity of contractions appear to be related to the height of the fever. Fetal distress is common, but frequently not diagnosed. The prognosis for the fetus is poor in severe disease.

Associated infections occur; pneumonia and urinary tract infections are common.

Management

- Pregnant women with severe malaria should be transferred to intensive care if possible.

- Monitoring of uterine contractions and fetal heart rate may reveal asymptomatic labour and fetal tachycardia, bradycardia, or late deceleration in relation to uterine contractions, indicating fetal distress.

- Once labour has started, fetal or maternal distress may indicate the need to shorten the second stage by forceps or vacuum extraction, or caesarean section.

Hypoglycaemia

Clinical features (see pages 17–18)

Hypoglycaemia may be present in pregnant women on admission, or may occur after quinine infusion. It is commonly asymptomatic, although it may be associated with fetal brady-cardia and other signs of fetal distress. In the most severely ill patients, it is associated with lactic acidosis and high mortality.

In patients who have been given quinine, abnormal behaviour, sweating, and sudden loss of consciousness are the usual manifestations.

Management

- Treat as described on page 18. If the diagnosis is in doubt, a therapeutic test with 50% glucose (25–50 ml intravenously) should be used.

- Recurrent severe hypoglycaemia may be a problem in some cases.

- If injectable glucose is not available, glucose solutions can be given to unconscious patients through a nasogastric tube.

Pulmonary oedema

Clinical features

Pulmonary oedema may be present in pregnant women on admission, may develop suddenly and unexpectedly several days after admission, or may develop immediately after childbirth (Fig. 10) (see also page 20).

Management

- Treat as described on page 21.

Anaemia

Clinical features (see page 15)

Maternal anaemia is associated with perinatal mortality, maternal morbidity and an increased risk of fatal maternal postpartum haemorrhage. A syndrome of acute severe haemolytic anaemia, especially in midpregnancy in women with splenomegaly, has been described in Africa.

Women who go into labour when severely anaemic or fluid-overloaded may develop pulmonary oedema after separation of the placenta.

Management

- Women with a haematocrit lower than 20% should receive a slow transfusion of packed cells (with the precautions mentioned on page 16) and furosemide 20 mg intravenously; alternatively, they may be given exchange transfusion (in centres where this can be done safely).

Antimalarial drugs

Chloroquine can be used safely in pregnancy. Quinine, in the doses advocated for the treatment of life-threatening malaria, is safe. It has been shown that the initial intravenous infusion of quinine in women who are more than 30 weeks pregnant is not associated with uterine stimulation or fetal distress. Its major adverse effect is hypoglycaemia. Mefloquine appears to be safe and effective in the treatment of uncomplicated falciparum malaria except in the first trimester and can be used as an adjunct to quinine infusion in severe malaria when the patient can take oral medication (see Table 1 inside front cover flap and Annex 1).

Diagnosis of malaria

Clinical diagnosis

The most important element in the clinical diagnosis of malaria, in both endemic and nonendemic areas, is to have a high index of suspicion.

Because the distribution of malaria is patchy, even in countries where it is known to be prevalent, a geographical and travel history indicative of exposure is important. In addition, the possibility of induced malaria (through transfusion or use of contaminated needles) must not be overlooked.

Severe malaria can mimic many other diseases that are also common in malarious countries. The most important of these are all types of meningitis, typhoid fever and septicaemia. Other differential diagnoses include influenza, hepatitis, leptospirosis, the relapsing fevers, haemorrhagic fevers, scrub typhus, all types of viral encephalitis, gastroenteritis and, in Africa, trypanosomiasis.

In pregnant women, malaria must be distinguished from sepsis arising in the uterus, urinary tract or breast.

In children, convulsions due to malaria must be differentiated from febrile convulsions. In the latter, coma rarely lasts for more than half an hour after the ictal phase.

Parasitological diagnosis

In the majority of cases, examination of thick and thin films of the peripheral blood will reveal malaria parasites. Thick films are more useful than thin films in the detection of malaria parasitaemia (Fig. 11 and 12). It is essential that facilities and

Fig. 11. Appearance of *P. falciparum* parasite stages in Giemsa-stained thin and thick blood films

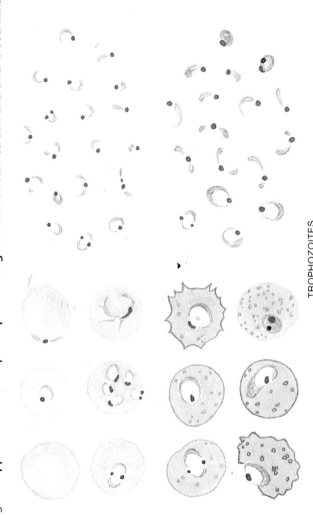

TROPHOZOITES

SCHIZONTS

GAMETOCYTES

Thick film

Thin film

Species		*Plasmodium falciparum*	*P. vivax*
		Young, growing trophozoites and/or mature gametocytes usually seen.	All stages seen; Schüffner's stippling in 'ghost' of host red cells, especially at film edge.
Stage of parasite in peripheral blood	Gametocyte	Immature pointed-end forms uncommon. *Mature forms*: banana-shaped or rounded; *chromatin*: single, well defined; *pigment*: scattered, coarse, rice-grain like; pink extrusion body sometimes present. Eroded forms with only chromatin and pigment often seen.	Immature forms difficult to distinguish from mature trophozoites. *Mature forms*: round, large; *chromatin*: single, well defined; *pigment*: scattered, fine. Eroded forms with scanty or no cytoplasm and only chromatin and pigment present.
	Schizont	Usually associated with many young ring forms. *Size*: small, compact; *number*: few, uncommon, usually in severe malaria; *mature forms*: 12–30 or more merozoites in compact cluster; *pigment*: single dark mass.	*Size*: large; *number*: few to moderate; *mature forms*: 12–24 merozoites, usually 16, in irregular cluster; *pigment*: loose mass.
	Trophozoite	*Size*: small to medium; *number*: often numerous; *shape*: ring and comma forms common; *chromatin*: often two dots; *cytoplasm*: regular, fine to fleshy; *mature forms*: sometimes present in severe malaria, compact with pigment as few coarse grains or a mass.	*Size*: small to large; *number*: few to moderate; *shape*: broken ring to irregular forms common; *chromatin*: single, occasionally two; *cytoplasm*: irregular or fragmented; *mature forms*: compact, dense; *pigment*: scattered, fine.

	P. ovale	*P. malariae*	
	All stages seen; prominent Schüffner's stippling in 'ghost' of host red cells, especially at film edge.	All stages seen.	

P. ovale column, top row (immature/mature forms): Immature forms difficult to distinguish from mature trophozoites. *Mature forms:* round, may be smaller than *P. vivax; chromatin:* single, well defined; *pigment:* scattered, coarse. Eroded forms with only chromatin and pigment present.

P. malariae column, top row: Immature and certain mature forms difficult to distinguish from mature trophozoites *Mature forms:* round, compact; *chromatin:* single, well defined; *pigment:* scattered, coarse, may be peripherally distributed. Eroded forms with only chromatin and pigment present.

P. ovale column, middle row: *Size:* rather like *P. malariae; number:* few; *mature forms:* 4–12 merozoites, usually 8, in loose cluster; *pigment:* concentrated mass.

P. malariae column, middle row: *Size:* small, compact; *number:* usually few; *mature forms:* 6–12 merozoites, usually 8, in loose cluster; some apparently without cytoplasm; *pigment:* concentrated.

P. ovale column, bottom row: *Size:* may be smaller than *P. vivax; number:* usually few; *shape:* ring to rounded, compact forms; *chromatin:* single, prominent; *cytoplasm:* fairly regular, fleshy; *pigment:* scattered, coarse.

P. malariae column, bottom row: *Size:* small; *number:* usually few; *shape:* ring to rounded, compact forms; *chromatin:* single, large; *cytoplasm:* scattered, regular, dense; *pigment:* scattered, abundant, with yellow tinge in older forms.

Fig. 12. **Species identification of malaria parasites in Giemsa-stained thick blood films**

equipment for microscopic examination of blood films are available; such examinations can be easily carried out by trained personnel in a side-room as well as in the laboratory.

Although occasional reports have described individuals dying from autopsy-proven cerebral malaria in whom there was no detectable peripheral parasitaemia, in the majority of patients with severe malaria high parasite counts are usually seen, unless the patient has already taken antimalarial drugs (this is becoming increasingly common in the tropics) or the infection is highly synchronous.

While high parasite densities can usually be equated with severe disease, the reverse is not always true. There may be wide differences between the number of parasitized cells in the peripheral blood and the number sequestered; moreover, rapid changes may be expected in synchronous infections. Frequent monitoring of the parasitaemia (every 4–6 hours) is very important for the first 2–3 days of treatment.

The presence of malaria pigment in monocytes is a useful indication of the diagnosis of malaria, especially in anaemic children and in patients with severe malaria associated with absent or low parasitaemia.

Haematological and biochemical findings

Thrombocytopenia is almost invariably present and peripheral leukocytosis is found in patients with the most severe disease. Elevation of serum urea, creatinine, bilirubin and enzymes, e.g. aminotransferases and 5'-nucleotidase may be found. Severely ill patients are acidotic, with low capillary plasma pH and bicarbonate concentrations. Fluid and electrolyte disturbances (sodium, potassium, chloride, calcium and phosphate) are variable. Concentrations of lactic acid in the blood and cerebrospinal fluid are high in both adults and children.

Prognostic indicators

The major indicators of a poor prognosis in children and adults with severe malaria are listed below.

Clinical indicators

Age under 3 years
Deep coma
Witnessed or reported convulsions
Absent corneal reflexes
Decerebrate rigidity (see Fig. 6)
Clinical signs of organ dysfunction (e.g. renal failure, pulmonary oedema)
Retinal haemorrhages (see Fig. 3).

Laboratory indicators

Hyperparasitaemia (>250 000/µl or >5%) (see page 25)
Peripheral schizontaemia (Fig. 11 and 12).
Peripheral leukocytosis (>12 000/µl)
Packed cell volume less than 20%
Haemoglobin less than 4.4 mmol/l (<7.1 g/dl)
Blood glucose less than 2.2 mmol/l (<40 mg/dl)
Blood urea more than 21.4 mmol/l (>60 mg of urea nitrogen per dl)
Low CSF glucose
Creatinine more than 265 µmol/l (>3.0 mg/dl)
High CSF lactic acid (>6 mmol/l)
Raised venous lactic acid (>6 mmol/l)
More than 3-fold elevation of serum enzymes (aminotransferases)
Increased plasma 5'-nucleotidase
Low antithrombin III levels

Common errors in diagnosis and management

The common errors in the diagnosis and management of severe malaria are listed below.

Errors in diagnosis

Failure to do a malarial blood film
Failure to take a travel history
Misjudgement of severity
Faulty parasitological diagnosis and laboratory management
Failure to diagnose other associated infections
Missed hypoglycaemia
Failure to carry out an ophthalmoscopic examination for the presence of retinal haemorrhages
Misdiagnosis (e.g. influenza, viral encephalitis, hepatitis, scrub typhus, etc.)

Errors in management

Inadequate nursing care (see page 9)
Errors of fluid and electrolyte replacement (see pages 18–19).
Delay in starting antimalarial therapy
Use of an inappropriate drug (e.g. chloroquine in areas of resistance)
Unjustified withholding of an antimalarial drug (see page 6)
Dosage not correctly calculated
Inappropriate route of administration (see front cover flap)
Failure to elicit a history of recent chemotherapy
Unjustified cessation of treatment
Failure to control the rate of intravenous infusion

Failure to prevent cumulative effects of antimalarial drugs

Failure to switch patients from parenteral to oral therapy as soon as they can take oral medication

Unnecessary continuation of chemotherapy beyond the recommended length of treatment (see front cover flap)

Unnecessary endotracheal intubation

Failure to prevent or control convulsions

Failure to recognize and treat severe anaemia

Use of potentially dangerous ancillary therapies (see page 15)

Delay in considering obstetrical intervention in late pregnancy

Failure to recognize and manage pulmonary oedema, aspiration pneumonia, and metabolic acidosis

Delay in starting peritoneal dialysis or haemodialysis

Failure to review antimalarial treatment in a patient whose condition is deteriorating

◼ **Selected further reading**

Basic malaria microscopy. Part I : Learner's guide. Part II: Tutor's guide. Geneva, World Health Organization, 1991.

Bench aids for the diagnosis of malaria. Plates No. 1-8. Geneva, World Health Organization, 1988.

International travel and health. Vaccination requirements and health advice. Geneva, World Health Organization (updated annually).

Warrell. D. A. et al., ed. Severe and complicated malaria, 2nd ed. *Transactions of the Royal Society of Tropical Medicine and Hygiene*, 84 (Suppl. 2): 1–65 (1990).

WHO model prescribing information: drugs used in parasitic diseases, 2nd edition ed. Geneva, World Health Organization, 1995

WHO Technical Report Series, No. 805, 1990 *(Practical chemotherapy of malaria:* report of a WHO Scientific Group).

Notes on antimalarial drugs

Quinine

At present, quinine remains the drug of choice for the treatment of severe and complicated malaria. It should always be given by rate-controlled infusion, **never** by bolus intravenous injection. Quinine is safe in pregnancy.

Mild side-effects are common, notably cinchonism (tinnitus, hearing loss, nausea, uneasiness, restlessness and blurring of vision); serious cardiovascular and neurological toxicity is rare. Hypoglycaemia is the most serious frequent adverse side-effect. In suspected quinine poisoning, activated charcoal given orally or by nasogastric tube accelerates elimination.

Chloroquine

Chloroquine is still the most widely prescribed antimalarial drug in the tropics. Despite parasite resistance, it provides symptomatic relief and reduces morbidity and mortality in many endemic areas where the resistance is predominantly RI or RII. In severe disease, chloroquine, like quinine, should always be given by slow rate-controlled intravenous infusion and **never** by bolus injection. It can also be given intramuscularly or subcutaneously at a lower dosage than that recommended for intravenous infusion. Oral therapy should be substituted as soon as possible; chloroquine can be given by nasogastric tube if injection is not possible. Immediate side-effects include nausea, vomiting, headache, uneasiness, restlessness, blurred vision, hypotension and pruritus. Acute chloroquine poisoning is manifested by coma, convulsions, dysrhythmias and hypotension.

Mefloquine

Mefloquine is effective against all malarial species including multidrug-resistant *P. falciparum*. Structurally, it resembles quinine. Naturally resistant parasite populations have been reported from various parts of the tropics. It is available only in tablet form. Toxic effects include nausea, abdominal discomfort, diarrhoea, vertigo, hypotension, and asymptomatic sinus arrhythmia and sinus bradycardia. Acute psychosis and a transient encephalopathy with convulsions are serious though relatively rare and short-lived side-effects.

Halofantrine

Halofantrine is a phenanthrenemethanol recently introduced into clinical practice. It is active against multidrug-resistant falciparum malaria; there is no parenteral preparation. Oral bioavailability (including absorption) of the drug is poor, but can be increased if the drug is taken with a fatty meal. Reported side-effects to date are very few — abdominal pain, diarrhoea and pruritus have been recorded. Halofantrine is not recommended for use in pregnancy.

Sulfadoxine–pyrimethamine (500 mg + 25 mg)

Sulfadoxine–pyrimethamine should preferably not be given in late pregnancy or to newborn infants because of the theoretical risk of provoking kernicterus. A painful intramuscular preparation exists and may be useful for treatment of severe malaria if chloroquine and quinine are not available, or if chloroquine is not effective. Severe reactions are rare when this drug combination is used as a single-dose treatment in the prescribed manner. Resistance is widespread.

Qinghaosu

Clinical trials to date of artemisinin and related compounds — artemether (intramuscular preparation) and artesunate (oral and intravenous preparations) — suggest that these compounds may be superior to the quinolone antimalarials for the treatment of both uncomplicated and complicated malaria. Their rapidity of action, relative safety to date, novel molecular structure and mode of action augur well for the future.

Annex 2

■ The Glasgow coma scale

		Score
Eyes open:	spontaneously	4
	to speech	3
	to pain	2
	never	1
Best verbal response:	oriented	5
	confused	4
	inappropriate words	3
	incomprehensible sounds	2
	none	1
Best motor response:	obeys commands	6
	localizes pain	5
	flexion to pain:	
	withdrawal	4
	abnormal	3
	extension to pain	2
	none	1
	Total	**3–15**

This score has been modified to be applicable to children, including those who have not learned to speak.

		Score
Eye movements:	directed (e.g. follows mother's face)	1
	not directed	0
Verbal response:	appropriate cry	2
	moan or inappropriate cry	1
	none	0
Best motor response:	localizes painful stimulus[a]	2
	withdraws limb from pain[b]	1
	nonspecific or absent response	0
	Total	**0–5**

These scales can be used repeatedly to assess improvement or deterioration.

[a] Rub knuckles on patient's sternum.
[b] Firm pressure on thumbnail bed with horizontal pencil.

Annex 3

■ Measurement of central
■ venous pressure

The jugular venous pressure is usually measured with the patient propped up at 45° to the horizontal. The venous pressure waves in the internal jugular vein become visible in the supraclavicular fossa (provided the neck muscles are relaxed) at a pressure of approximately 4 cm H_2O. The wave form is characteristic in sinus rhythm (two waves for every arterial pulse). The height of the wave relative to the clavicles can be increased by lowering the patient, and the wave itself is usually not palpable. It must be distinguished from the carotid arterial pulsation. Measurement of the central venous pressure by examination of the external jugular vein or the filling of veins on the dorsum of the hand at different arm elevations is less reliable (e.g. the external jugular vein may be kinked in the supraclavicular fossa, and therefore not in free communication with the great veins and right atrium). However, rapid emptying of neck veins distended by occluding them at the base of the neck indicates that the venous pressure is not high.

In seriously ill patients, or those in whom assessment is considered inaccurate, a central venous catheter should be inserted. The catheter may be inserted into the jugular or subclavian vein provided that adequate facilities for a sterile procedure and subsequent nursing are available. Four approaches are possible: antecubital (Fig. A3.1), infraclavicular (Fig. A3.2), internal jugular and supraclavicular (Fig. A3.3).

Before readings can be taken, the zero on the manometer must be aligned as accurately as possible with the horizontal plane of the right atrium. A simple spirit level (e.g. 20-ml glass ampoule containing liquid with a bubble, taped to a ruler) can

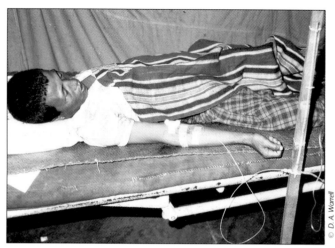

Fig. A3.1.

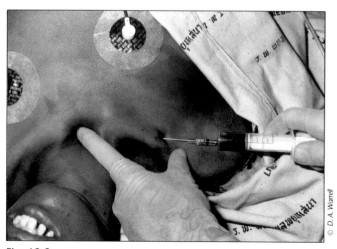

Fig. A3.2.

Fig. A3.1. Central venous pressure monitoring in a township hospital in rural Myanmar (Burma). A 70-cm catheter was inserted into an antecubital vein (Seldinger technique) and advanced until its tip was in the superior vena cava. An extension tube is connected to a simple saline manometer with its zero point at the level of the mid-axillary line

Fig. A3.2. Central venous pressure monitoring. Puncture of the subclavian vein (infraclavicular approach) preparatory to inserting a guide wire and short catheter (Seldinger technique)

Fig. A3.3. Central venous pressure monitoring. Surface markings of the subclavian vein for needle insertion by the supraclavicular approach

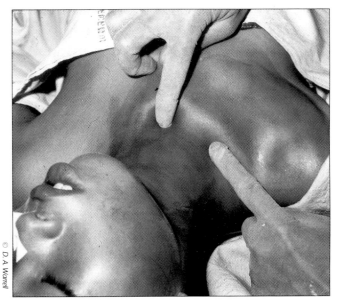

© D. A. Warrell

Fig. A3.3.

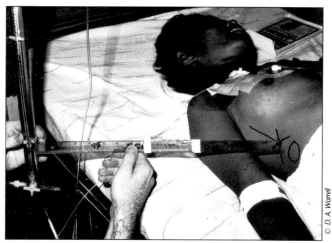

© D. A. Warrell

Fig. A3.4. **Levelling of the central venous pressure manometer at the mid-axillary line using a home-made
spirit level (ruler plus glass ampoule), in a Thai
provincial hospital**

be used to locate the manometer zero at the same height as an
appropriate chest-wall landmark, such as the mid-axillary line,
in the supine patient (Fig. A3.4).

If a central venous catheter is used, strict attention must be
given to asepsis. Infection, air embolism and thrombosis are
potential complications, especially if the catheter remains in
place for a long time.